Hydrogen Peroxide Miracles & Cures Handbook

Benefits, Uses & Medical Therapy with Hydrogen Peroxide

Table of Contents

Copyright 2015 by Greg Cook - All rights reserved.

Introduction

Thank you for purchasing this book entitled *"Hydrogen Peroxide Miracles & Cures Handbook: Benefits, Uses & Medical Therapy with Hydrogen Peroxide"*.

From this book, you will find proven steps and strategies on how to use and benefit from hydrogen peroxide as:

- Natural antibiotic to treat infections

- Solution to protect and maintain dental health

- Adjunct treatment for cancer

- Natural product for personal and skin care

- Natural remedy to treat various diseases, health conditions, and disorders such as nasal congestion, nail fungus, dry skin, canker sores, acne breakouts, toothache, head lice, yeast infections, and body odor

- Effective and affordable solution to promote a home environment free from bad bacteria

- Natural remedy to protect the health of your pets

You will also get to know more about the wonder that is hydrogen peroxide and how it can save you your hard-earned money as you enjoy all its benefits. Use this book as your friendly guide and see how you will be able to improve the way you deal with certain health conditions simply by benefiting from hydrogen peroxide.

Again, thank you for purchasing this book.

Chapter 1: All That You Need to Know About Hydrogen Peroxide

Hydrogen peroxide, whose chemical formula is H_2O_2, is a popular disinfectant commonly used in clinics and hospitals. Clinical personnel use it to cleanse and disinfect wounds. However, there is more to H_2O_2 than just its popular use. In this chapter, you'll get to know more about this chemical compound that works wonder.

Chemical Formula

If you look at the formula of hydrogen peroxide, it closely resembles that of the chemical formula for water: H_2O_2 (hydrogen peroxide) vs. H_2O (water). The only difference is that there is extra oxygen in hydrogen peroxide, hence the subscript "2" in the formula.

Unlike water which is a very stable compound, hydrogen peroxide is less stable. It decomposes into oxygen and water. The decomposition, though, happens really slowly that it becomes negligible.

However, since it is unstable, H2O2 is sensitive to sunlight and heat. Thus, you should store it in a place where temperature is below 30°C and where it can avoid exposure to sunlight. Its instability is also the reason H_2O_2 comes in dark-colored bottles.

Grades or Strengths

In buying hydrogen peroxide, it matters that you are aware of its different grades, concentrations, or strengths. Use the following table as your quick reference:

3.0-3.5 %	**Pharmaceutical grade-** the kind that you will find readily available over the counter at drugstores and supermarkets. However, you should not use this internally as it contains stabilizers that can be toxic when ingested.
35%	**Food grade** – is safe for ingestion. Manufacturers usually use this for producing commercially available food such as eggs, cheese, and products that contain whey. They also use this to spray the foil lining of milk and fruit juice packages.

35%	**Technical grade** – highly concentrated, this is meant for hot tubs and as a sterilizing agent.
30%	**Reagent grade** - contains stabilizers not safe for ingestion. The most common use is for scientific experiments.
30-32%	**Electronic grade** – is suitable to clean electronic gadget parts.
6%	**Beautician/Cosmetic grade** – commonly used as a hair bleaching agent. In beauty parlors, you will see hydrogen peroxide being used as a liquid developer to color hair.

In this handbook, the hydrogen peroxide that you will mostly need is either the 35% food grade or the 3.5% pharmaceutical grade.

Precautionary Measures

Here are some precautionary measures to observe, irrespective of how safe hydrogen peroxide is. Remember that the discussion presented in this handbook revolves around two grades: (1) pharmaceutical grade that you can buy easily from any of these sources: online stores, your local drugstores, and the supermarkets; and (2) food grade which you can also buy online or from your drugstores.

Between the two grades, however, only the 35% food grade is safe for ingestion. You should never attempt to take the 3.5% pharmaceutical grade internally, as it is strictly for external use only.

Diluting 35% Food Grade

Often, it is best to dilute the 35% food grade H_2O_2 into either 3% solution or 6% solution. Observe the following when diluting:

- Use distilled water only for the dilution. As mentioned earlier, hydrogen peroxide is unstable and may lose its strength and decomposes when in contact with other substances such as water impurities and minerals.

- Distilled water is free from these impurities and other substances that may react with H_2O_2 upon contact. Aside from pure water, you also need to make sure to use a container that is clean and hygienic.

- For your own protection, wear gloves for your hands and goggles for your eyes. As much as possible, avoid the solution to come in contact with your hands, skin, and eyes.   If it does, wash it right away with lots of water.

- The recommended ratio to follow to dilute:

	Hydrogen Peroxide (35% Food Grade)	Distilled Water
3% Solution	1 Part	11 Parts
6% Solution	2 Parts	11 Parts

In some countries like the UK, you may no longer purchase hydrogen peroxide in concentrations 12+ % unless you have a license to purchase such. The limit for ordinary consumers is 12% and below.

It is best to dilute the 35% food grade if you plan to consume it internally.   Make sure that what you will use is high quality H_2O_2 food grade.

Two things to follow strictly:

1. Handle the peroxide with strict care and avoid any contact with your skin and eyes.   Wear protection such as hand gloves and goggles.

2. Store your diluted peroxide in appropriate container and store it in a place away from heat and light.

Chapter 2:   How Hydrogen Peroxide Allows You to Save Your Hard-earned Money

One of the most notable benefits of using hydrogen peroxide is that it can save you from spending your hard-earned money from costly treatments.   In this chapter, you'll find out how to use this colorless liquid as a natural remedy that is not only safe but is also gentle on your pocket.

Natural Antibiotic

Hydrogen peroxide (H_2O_2) works as safe alternative to drug-based antibiotics.   In fact, it is one of the best natural remedies to fight infections prior to pharmaceutical antibiotics. Now that people are clamoring for safer alternatives due to issues with antibiotic use, H_2O_2 is fast regaining its popularity, which it rightfully deserves.

Three things why you should consider using hydrogen peroxide as a natural antibiotic:

1. It is generally safe that allows you to avoid the side effects common to drug-based antibiotics. The two main components of hydrogen peroxide are water and oxygen and none of

the synthetic chemicals common to pharmaceutical antibiotics.

2. You can easily and readily buy it from online stores, local pharmacies or drugstores, and supermarkets.

3. It is one of the most versatile natural remedies. Its use is not limited to treating infections.

If you're wondering how hydrogen peroxide works as an antibiotic, consider the following:

- Once this colorless liquid comes in contact with your body or skin, it releases its oxygen that destroys bacteria. Clinical studies have also shown that H_2O_2 can stop and inhibit viruses, parasites, and fungi. It has also demonstrated its ability to rescind certain tumors when administered intravenously.

- When H_2O_2 breaks into its elements- water and oxygen, the extra oxygen present in the formula creates an environment in your body that is hostile to pathogens. Thus, it denies and drives away these pathogens while restoring your body's good health condition and wellness.

Dental Health

Another way you can save lots of money with hydrogen peroxide is to use it to maintain your good dental health condition. Undeniably, maintaining your oral health can take much from your budget. Using hydrogen peroxide is one effective solution to stay on budget without compromising you dental health.

Look at what hydrogen peroxide can do for your dental health:

- It can stop and prevent the formation of plaque in your gums and teeth, thus, enabling you to avoid gum diseases such as gingivitis, periodontitis, abscesses, and lesions, as well as tooth decay.

- It prevents pathogens to invade your mouth causing gum and teeth infections, which otherwise can be very expensive to treat. This is because the chemical formula of hydrogen peroxide encourages anti-microbial activity in your mouth that drives the pathogens away.

Aside from these dental health benefits, H_2O_2 also works as an effective and low-cost teeth whitening agent. If you want to enjoy your pearly whites minus the cost, it's about time you consider benefiting from hydrogen peroxide.

Cancer Treatment

Inarguably, cancer is an extremely costly disease. Unfortunately, cancer has also grown as one of the most prevalent diseases today. It can hit anyone regardless of age, gender, race, or financial status in life.

If cancer has hit anyone in your family, you can reduce the cost of treatment by benefiting from hydrogen peroxide treatment. However, H2O2 is neither a complete treatment for cancer nor is it able to reverse the damage of cancer to your healthy cells (such as those who have undergone medical treatment like chemotherapy).

What it can do most effectively is to prevent cancer cells to spread and to promote the formation of healthy cells in the body. Thus, this treatment is most beneficial to individuals who are in their early stages of cancer and to those who have not yet undergone aggressive treatment for cancer.

In consideration of the aforementioned, it is best to use it as an adjunct treatment to boost your recommended primary treatment for cancer. This way, you do not only increase the chances of reversing the disease safely without the usual side effects, but you can also save much on the cost of the cancer treatment.

How does hydrogen peroxide heal cancer? Studies reveal that cancer cells thrive in an environment where glucose (sugar) is bountiful and oxygen is scarce. These cells metabolize sugar without needing oxygen; the reason cancer craves for sugar but hates oxygen. Thus, supplying the body with pure oxygen can help in inhibiting the formation of cancer cells by denying them the environment they need to thrive.

Another essential thing to consider in using H2O2 as part of cancer treatment is the quality or purity of the solution. The only hydrogen peroxide you should use is the one labeled as food grade. Typically, your health practitioner will administer high quality food grade H2O2 intravenously.

While apparently there is no issue regarding the administration of H2O2 intravenously or externally, the controversy is in consuming it orally. To make it clear, health experts agree that only food grade hydrogen peroxide is suitable for internal consumption, but they also differ in their views on how safe it is for oral consumption.

For those who have advised against its oral consumption such as Robert O. Young, PhD, they argue that there is an increased risk of intestinal damage when H2O2 combines with or reacts to other substances or chemicals in the body such as superoxide.

Contrariwise, those who recommend its oral consumption assert its safeness. Dr. David G. Williams, from his laborious research concludes that while hydrogen peroxide in reaction to other chemicals may convert into free radical, the human body has the ability to use the free radical to destroy pathogens such as bacteria, fungi, and viruses.

Further Dr. Williams emphasizes how the body actually creates hydrogen peroxide necessary for white blood cells to do its job of protecting the system from pathogenic invasion, infections, and other culprits. Nevertheless, limit the oral consumption of hydrogen peroxide to the treatment of cancer, and avoid consuming it internally for other purposes or for maintaining your general health condition.

Multi Remedy

Hydrogen peroxide can treat multiple health conditions that normally require costly medications. Most of these conditions are either precursor to more serious diseases or they are life threatening themselves.
Look at this list of health conditions that H2O2 therapy can treat successfully:
- Emphysema

- Arrhythmia Influenza
- Liver Cirrhosis from Bacterial Infections
- Candida Parasitic Infections
- Parkinson's Disease
- Type 2 Diabetes
- Rheumatoid Arthritis
- Food Allergies
- Fungal and Yeast Infections
- Bacterial Infections
- Herpes Simplex
- Herpes Zoster
- Cerebral Vascular Disease
- Cardiovascular Disease
- Periodontal Disease
- Upper Respiratory Infections

Personal Care

You can do away with many expensive personal care products and substitute them with hydrogen peroxide, such as with the following:

- Teeth Whiteners – you can skip the dental strips to whiten your teeth and benefit from H2O2 instead. You just have to make sure that you do not have silver amalgam fillings to avoid reaction such as fumes.

- Tooth Paste – when mixed with baking soda, hydrogen peroxide can work as your natural tooth paste. Health experts find this solution as a heathier option than commercial toothpastes.

- Facial Toner – replace your usual toner brand with hydrogen peroxide solution to give you clearer skin. It can also get rid of acne from bacterial infections and prevent excessive oil on your face.

- Anti-Dandruff Rinse – when mixed with apple cider vinegar (ACV) and distilled water, H2O2 works to get rid and control dandruff. One major cause of dandruff is the overgrowth of yeas which hydrogen peroxide along with ACV can handle effectively with safe results.

Chapter 3: Steps and Procedures on How to Use Hydrogen Peroxide

This chapter serves as your easy reference on how to use hydrogen peroxide for its many health benefits as well as other benefits. You will find that the steps and procedures are simple. You just have to keep in mind that you will use-depending on your purpose, only the food grade and the pharmaceutical grade H2O2. Thus, forget about the other grades and focus on these two.

Treating Nasal Congestion

Nasal congestion usually occurs with common colds and flu. It can be very inconvenient and sometimes painful to have. To decongest, here's how to use 3% hydrogen peroxide:

1. Prepare the things you will use to treat nasal congestion: 3% hydrogen peroxide, tissue paper, pillow, and cotton swab.

2. Open the bottle of hydrogen peroxide and pour some into its cap to soak the cotton swab.

3. Tilt your head as you lay on the pillow. Slowly insert the cotton swab into just the opening of your ear (never insert the swab inside your ear). Squeeze the end of the

swab to release h2O2 up to two droplets. You may need to re-soak the swab to release another set of two droplets into your ear.

4. Stay in this position for about five minutes. It is normal to hear bubbling sound as this only means the peroxide is releasing its elements, water and oxygen, that will destroy the pathogen causing you your nasal congestion.

5. After five minutes, move your head back to its normal position. Using tissue paper, wipe any excess liquid that may drip from your ear. Repeat steps #3-5 to cover your other ear.

This procedure is best for young adults to adults. Avoid applying this to kids, as they may react differently to the bubbling sound.

Nail Fungus Remover

H2O2 works effectively to remove nail fungus. Here's how to do it:

<u>Single Nail Fungal Infection</u>

1. Wash the infected nail with mild soap and rinse it off with warm water. Dry the nail completely.

2.   Pour enough amount of hydrogen peroxide to soak the center of a cotton pad (you may also use cotton ball).   Place the H_2O_2-soaked pad onto the affected nail. Let the pad stay for five minutes.

3.   Remove the pad and dry the nail with a clean pad or a tissue. Do this procedure three times a day until the fungus disappears.

Multiple Nail Fungal Infection

1.   Use a basin where you can soak your hand/s or feet accordingly.   Fill the basin with sufficient warm water for soaking.   Follow this ratio to create your hydrogen peroxide solution: 1 part water: 1 part 3% H_2O_2.

2.   For severe fungal infection, you may add apple cider vinegar (ACV) into the solution following this ratio: 1 part water: 1 part 3% H_2O_2: 1 part ACV.

3.   Soak your hands or feet for 15-30 minutes. Rinse off with warm water.   Dry your hands or feet with a clean towel.   Repeat the procedure two to three times daily until the infection is gone or do it nightly for six (6) weeks.

Heal Dry Skin

If you have dry skin, you can benefit much from hydrogen peroxide therapy. With the therapy, you can prevent your dry skin to progress into eczema.

Follow these steps:

1. Add about ½ pint of hydrogen peroxide (diluted food grade solution) to your warm bath water. Make sure that it mixes well with the water before you soak your body.

2. Soak and relax your body in the tub for about 15-25 minutes. You have option to follow these up with a gentle scrub to exfoliate dead skin cells. Further, you may add any of the following into the solution: Epsom salt, herbal infusion, or essential oil.

3. Dry yourself thoroughly with a clean towel. Repeat this procedure for seven consecutive days to heal your dry skin. You may also do this once a month as a preventive measure.

Canker Sore Treatment

If your canker sore is causing you pain and discomfort, instead of waiting it to go away on its own, speed up the healing process with H2O2. Use the diluted solution discussed in Chapter 1 especially if you need to use the solution as your mouthwash.

Two ways to relieve the pain and discomfort those canker sores bring using 3% H2O2 diluted solution:

1. Apply the solution directly onto the sore.

2. Use the solution to as a mouth rinse.

Direct Application

1. Wash the affected area with mild soap and water.   Dry with a clean towel.

2. Wet a cotton pad with the H2O2 solution and then apply it directly onto the sore.

3. Repeat this procedure three times daily.

Mouth Rinse

1. After brushing your teeth, replace your usual mouthwash with the H2O2 solution. Swish for about a minute or two careful not to swallow the solution.
2. Rinse as necessary or at least three times daily until the sore goes away.

Clear and Prevent Acne

To clear and prevent acne breakouts, follow these steps:

1. Wash your face with a mild facial cleanser appropriate for your skin type. Dry with a clean facial towel.

2. Soak a cotton pad (cotton ball may substitute the pad) in 3% h2O2 solution. Apply it onto your face. Gently rub and massage the affected area with it.

3. Let the solution stay on your face for about five (5) minutes, after which rinse your face. Pat dry before your moisturize.

   Make sure to use the diluted solution (3%) and test it first onto your skin to check any reaction. If there is none, proceed with the aforementioned steps. Start with a weekly regimen (once a week application) and up to three times a week until the acne clears.

Toothache Solution

You would never want a toothache, as it is one of the most discomforting and painful conditions you could experience. While H_2O_2 does not directly relieve your pain and discomfort from toothache, it helps in getting rid of the cause by killing the pathogens that have invaded your gums and teeth.

Here are the steps to treat toothache with the solution:

1. Brush your teeth. Gargle with the H_2O_2 solution.

2. Following the gargling and rinsing of your mouth, apply the following:

    - Cold compress – for toothache from tooth decay, inflamed gums, or abscesses.

- Hot compress – for toothache from TMJ (temporomandibular joint) disorders

Teeth Whitener

If you wish to whiten your teeth with H2O2, follow these steps:

1. Check the ingredients of your regular toothpaste to see if it contains H2O2. You may have to switch brands if your current brand does not carry a whitening variant.

2. Create your H2O2 teeth whitening paste:

   Prepare the following:

   - Food grade hydrogen peroxide diluted into 3% solution, aluminum-free baking soda, mint oil (optional).

   - Mix hydrogen peroxide and baking soda well. Pour a few drops of mint oil to boost the bacteria-fighting properties of H2O2 as well as to add some flavor into your paste.

- Brush your teeth using your H_2O_2 toothpaste. Be careful not to swallow any residue when you rinse your mouth. You may also swish H_2O_2 solution as a mouth rinse. Follow this up by rinsing your mouth with pure water to H_2O_2 traces or residues.

Head Lice Treatment

Instead of using chemical-based head lice remover, benefit from the use of H_2O_2 solution.

Here's how:

1. Create your head lice remover by following this recipe:
2. Mix one part of 3% H_2O_2 with two parts of distilled water.

3. Pour the H_2O_2 mixture onto your scalp and start to massage the scalp with your fingers.

4. Without rinsing the mixture, cover your head with a clean towel. Let the mixture

stay on your scalp and hair for an hour or two.

5. Shampoo your hair (preferably choose one with coconut oil) and then rinse thoroughly.

Ridding Candida Albicans

Get rid of infections caused by Candida Albicans, such as vaginal yeast infection, with the following steps:

1. Create your own vaginal yeast home remedy by combining one part of 3% H_2O_2 with two parts of distilled water.

2. Apply the solution onto the affected area or use it as a vaginal rinse (do not douche).

Prevent Body Odor

You can prevent body odor without risking your skin to discoloration. Simply substitute your usual deodorant with H_2O_2 natural solution that you can do yourself. The added benefit is that you'll also be able to enjoy whiter underarms.

Here's how:

1. Dilute your food grade H_2O_2 into 3% solution. You may add essential oils for fragrance and to enhance the anti-bacterial properties of H_2O_2.
2. Apply the diluted solution onto your underarms.

Chapter 4: Other Incredible Uses and Benefits of Hydrogen Peroxide

You will love how hydrogen peroxide is a multi-purpose natural solution. In this chapter, you'll find out how to use it in your home and as part of your pet care remedies.

Vomit Inducer

If for any reason your pet has ingested something bad for their health, you can use H2O2 to induce vomiting. However, make sure that you call your pet's veterinarian right away. The H2O2 solution is just part of the first aid treatment, while waiting for the veterinary to apply the best treatment for your pet's condition.

In creating your H2O2 vomit inducer, mix one part of diluted food grade H2O2 (3% solution) with one part of distilled water. Administer one teaspoon of the mixture to your pet orally. Use a medicine dropper or a syringe as necessary.

Parasite Exterminator

To help clear parasites from your pet's skin, follow these steps:

1. Wash your pet using a natural soap preferably containing Gliricidia or Madre Cacao as ingredient. Another option is to use sulfur soap.

2. Rinse to remove the traces of soap. Follow this up with the H2O2 solution. Combine one part of H2O2 (3% solution) with two parts of warm water. Let the solution stay on your pet's skin for about 10 minutes.

3. Rinse with fresh water. Dry the skin of your pet and apply coconut oil to restore moisture and to prevent dryness of skin.

Natural Cleanser

Limit the use of chemical-based cleansers in your household to prevent toxins from entering your body through your skin or through inhalation. Use hydrogen peroxide-based cleansers as a healthy substitute. Here's how to create your natural cleanser:

Ingredients are as follows:

Floor Cleaner

- One cup of 3% pharmaceutical grade hydrogen peroxide
- One gallon of water

Just mix the two ingredients and start using it to clean the floor.

Anti-Bacterial Cleanser

- 3% pharmaceutical grade hydrogen peroxide
- Distilled water
- Apple cider vinegar

- Mix one part of H_2O_2 with one part of distilled water. Use this mixture together with apple cider vinegar simultaneously to kill bacteria such as E.coli and Salmonella.

Avoid mixing H2O2 with ACV to preserve both of their anti-bacterial properties. What you can do is to spray the area with the H2O2 solution first, then follow up with ACV, or you may also do the reverse-start with the ACV and end with the H2O2 solution.

Denture Cleaner

Commercial cleaners for dentures can be costly considering that you have to use it regularly. You can create your own natural denture cleanser by following these steps:

1. Mix one part of 3% diluted food grade hydrogen peroxide with two parts of distilled water. The amount should be enough to soak your dentures.

2. Brush your dentures with aluminum-free baking soda. Rinse it thoroughly with fresh water.

3. In a jar filled with the H_2O_2 solution, immerse your dentures. Close the lid and let your dentures soak for at least 15 minutes. You may also soak your dentures overnight, but be sure to replace the solution every day.

4. Before wearing your dentures, see to it that you rinse it off thoroughly with clean fresh water to remove any traces of H_2O_2.

Mold Remover

To remove molds that can stain and damage surfaces, use hydrogen peroxide solution. Here are the steps:

1. You will need the following materials: 3% pharmaceutical grade hydrogen peroxide, sponge, spray bottle, and cloth.

2. Fill your spray bottle with the 3% H2O2 solution and start spraying the mold with it. Allow the solution to sit for 15 minutes for the peroxide to do its job. Upon contact with the mold, you will see and hear the bubbling of the solution, which means that the H2O2 is releasing its properties to kill the bacteria.

3. After 15 minutes, wipe the surface with a damp cloth to remove the mold. Repeat this in all affected areas until you have gotten rid of all the molds.

4. Wash the area with soapy water and then rinse off. Let natural air dry the area, or alternatively use clean dry cloth to wipe the surfaces.

Fruit and Vegetable Rinse

Rinse your fruits and vegetables with H2O2 solution to remove traces of chemicals such as pesticides and fertilizers. Here's how:

1. Fill your spray bottle with 3% hydrogen peroxide solution. Fill another spray bottle with apple cider vinegar.

2. Wash your fruits and veggies in running water. Spray them with H2O2 and ACV in any order you wish.

3. Rinse your fruits and veggies in running water for about one minute.

Conclusion

Hydrogen peroxide or H2O2 is a natural solution that works wonders and miraculously. It has multiple benefits, such as:

Protecting your health and that of your family's health including your pets

Ensuring that your household is free from bacteria, viruses, parasites, and other pathogens that can increase your risks of diseases and infections

Allowing you to save on cost of drug-based treatments as well as household cleaners thereby protecting your budget from overshoots

As you have learned and realized from this book, to benefit much from the hydrogen peroxide solution, you need to use the right grade. For the benefits presented in this book, the required grade is either the food grade H2O2 or the pharmaceutical grade H2O2.

As a reminder, before using the food grade peroxide, you must dilute it first to arrive at a 3% solution. Otherwise, you run the risk of burns and other damages to your skin and health. You will also note that some countries like the UK are implementing regulations such as prohibiting the purchase of 35% food grade hydrogen peroxide unless the buyer has the necessary license. You should comply with these regulations, as applicable.

This book has also listed precautionary measures in using hydrogen peroxide. These measures are meant to give you the best experience and benefits in using the solution for whatever purpose you find it most appropriate.

When used properly, you have a miraculous solution that will protect your health, your family, your pet, and your home without hurting your pocket. Are you going to pass on this great opportunity?

Bonus Content

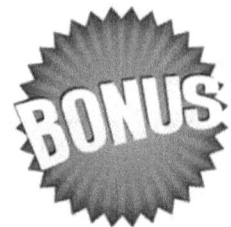

As a token of our appreciation Grand Reveur Publications would like to give you access to our exclusive bonus content (including free eBooks!).

Exclusive pre-release access to our latest eBooks Free Grand Reveur eBooks during promotional periods.

A method ANYONE can use to publish their own book and make passive income.

To receive this bonus content go to the following website:

https://ignorelimits.leadpages.net/grandreveur publications/

As this is a limited time offer it would be a shame to miss out, I recommend grabbing these bonuses before reading on.